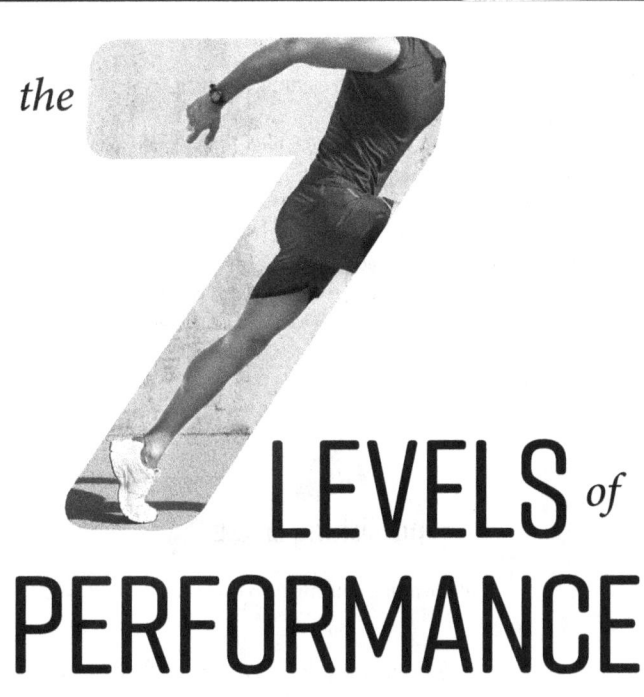

the 7 LEVELS of PERFORMANCE

THE ATHLETE'S
PLAYBOOK
FOR GETTING
IN THE ZONE

CHRIS MORGAN

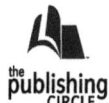

COPYRIGHT © 2017 CHRIS MORGAN

All rights reserved. No part of this publication may be reproduced, distributed or transmitted in any form or by any means, including photocopying, recording, or other electronic or mechanical methods, without the prior written permission of the publisher, except in the case of brief quotations embodied in critical reviews and certain other noncommercial uses permitted by copyright law. For permission requests, write to the publisher, addressed "Attention: Permissions Coordinator," at the address below.

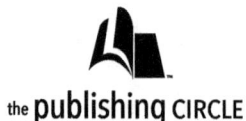

admin@ThePublishingCircle.com

or

THE PUBLISHING CIRCLE, LLC
Regarding: Chris Morgan
1603 Capitol Avenue
Suite 310
Cheyenne, Wyoming 82001

The publisher is not responsible for the author's website, other mentioned websites, or content of any website that is not owned by the publisher.

THE 7 LEVELS OF PERFORMANCE: THE ATHLETE'S PLAYBOOK FOR GETTING IN THE ZONE / CHRIS MORGAN – FIRST EDITION
ISBN 978-1-947398-00-9

Table of Contents

PART I: The Zone — 1

   CHAPTER 1 — 3
   The Seven Levels of Performance

   CHAPTER 2 — 12
   The Zone

   CHAPTER 3 — 21
   Getting in the Zone: The Mindset

   CHAPTER 4 — 31
   Getting in the Zone: Skill Development

PART II: Staying in the Zone — 43

   CHAPTER 5 — 45
   Zone Inhibitor: Fear and Worry

   CHAPTER 6 — 52
   Zone Inhibitor: Loss

   CHAPTER 7 — 56
   Zone Inhibitor: Injury

   CHAPTER 8 — 63
   Zone Inhibitor: Losing Motivation

   CHAPTER 9 — 69
   The Seven Levels of Performance Process

REFERENCES — 73

Author Biography

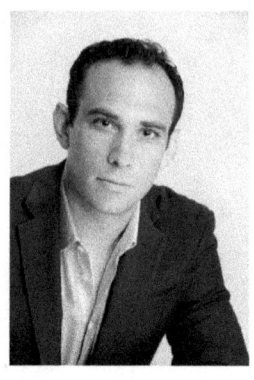

CHRIS MORGAN is a performance strategist, having dedicated the past 10 years of his life to working with teams to elevate their performance.

When he was competing as an athlete, Chris found that while sometimes he could get into peak states, it was hard to do this on a consistent basis. Often he found that the resulting dry spells in his performances would affect his personal life

However, when he learned about getting in the zone as a coach, Chris realized he could also help athletes with getting in the zone more consistently so that they could have their best performances.

Chris is sought out to help players for professional teams to breakthrough to higher levels of performance.

He lives in Alameda, California, and is an avid martial artist (Brazilian Jiu Jitsu), and runner.

www.ChrisMorganLive.com

*To all who strive
to be the champion in their sport,
and for the invisible championship
that is mastery of life.*

PART I

THE ZONE

The first part of this book is about the coveted, but seemingly elusive, "Zone State." The zone is the edge that all athletes look for in their careers. Learning more about it is to your advantage.

In this part, you will learn about the Seven Levels of Performance, which provides insight and guidance into the different mindsets you can adopt in any athletic pursuit (and life), and which will help you get into the zone. You will also learn more about the zone scientifically, how to trigger yourself into the zone, and how to approach training with the right mindset.

chapter

1

The Seven Levels of Performance

*"Good, better, best. Never let it rest,'
til your good is better and better is best."*
ST. JEROME

MOST OF YOUR ATHLETIC TRAINING (time and money) is likely spent on skills and conditioning coaching. That makes sense because of how critical proper skills and conditioning are for your success; but what about the mind game?

Performance is up to ninety percent mental (or, you can say it's ten percent mental but that ten percent controls all physical performance). However, do you give mindset development the appropriate amount of training and investment given its power over your performance?

My guess is that you probably do give mindset training some amount of attention. You are likely mentally strong already, and looking to improve and achieve that edge.

Getting in the zone consistently definitely provides an edge. Perhaps the edge. It involves mental toughness but ends up going well beyond it due to the biological properties of the zone that make your performance seem effortless, timeless, creative, and plain amazing (more on this in chapter two). Usually, you will perform at your absolute best when you are in the zone.

Performing at your best is what consistently makes legends. Whether you are an established professional, an aspiring professional, or a hobbyist, consistently performing is crucial to achieving your goals (e.g. a winning record, a championship, your legacy, your salary, your notoriety, and your career beyond athletics). The zone state can give you an edge in all of these aspects.

The zone state can seem so elusive. You likely have experienced it at least once before. Perhaps several times. However, you want to experience it on a consistent basis. How do you do this? How do you take control of your mindset to get in the zone as often as possible?

This book aims to demystify mindset and the results you obtain from the mindsets you are using in your sport. To be precise, they provide an understanding and pathway to experiencing the seemingly elusive zone state that you want to experience to achieve your optimal level performances.

On Mindset

The mind is quite possibly the most powerful gift bestowed upon us by our creator. With it, the most amazing inventions have been conceived of, and the most incredible athletic performances have been achieved. Any acts that we want to create, any accomplishment we want to achieve, begins in the mind. No other part of the human body has so much power.

To understand the mind is to gain power over your performances.

The mind can be broken down into two elements. The first is the brain, which controls your body's movements and functions, while storing information. It's where all of your habits, skills and routines lie. Your voluntary and involuntary responses travel through the nervous system. Once a skill or activity becomes second nature, it slips into your subconscious mind.

There's an incredible amount of research being done on the brain because it's such an amazing organ; it houses over 100 million neurons.[1] Nonetheless, the primary focus of this book will be on mindset development.

The second part is your consciousness or mindset. Bruce D Schneider, founder of the Institute for Professional Excellence in Coaching (iPEC), defines consciousness as "The level of your self-awareness, how fully you realize your true self, as opposed to the self you have been 'trained' to see and accept."[2]

Mindset determines how you summon your capabilities (skill and will) for your sport. It also allows you to re-program behavioral patterns that may have become ingrained over your lifetime. Sometimes these patterns serve you and your desire to experience peak performance in your sport; but more often than not, these patterns get in the way (e.g. fear and worry).

For instance, imagine you are a basketball player who gets upset at a referee who makes a call you do not agree with. You then become so angry that you receive a technical foul, or you are ejected from the game. This occurs because you are experiencing a behavioral pattern where you are not consciously controlling your mindset. Instead, you are letting your programming take its course.

Focus is the tool that allows you to shift your mindset. If your focus is on your defects, then many of your thought patterns will start manifesting and jeopardizing peak performance. When you start seeing yourself as having intrinsic value, maybe because you see yourself as being created in the image of God, or you just believe in your worth, then thought patterns begin to emerge that support peak performance.

By consciously choosing where to direct your focus, you can change your reaction to a response. For instance, you may focus more on the fact that there are an abundance of opportunities that you can capitalize on just waiting for you to spot them. Letting go of the referee call (which you can't control) would allow you to capitalize on these opportunities. This change in focus then provides a powerful shift in your mindset. The shift in mindset then allows you to perform at a much more efficient level.

So what is the basis of your mindset? Thoughts comprise the primary driver of your mindset. Thoughts, in turn, fuel the emotions you experience. Thoughts and emotions, in turn, produce your actions.

iPEC provides a useful model that summarizes the relationship of your thought-emotion-action-result[3]:

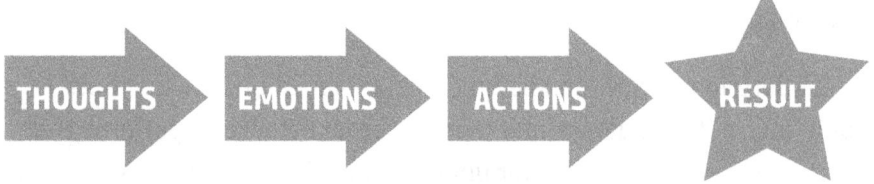

A thought is like a seed. If properly watered and exposed to sunlight, a seed grows into a mature plant. Your thoughts, if nourished, produce full results in your life. Emotions and actions are like the water and sunshine given to thoughts that are planted. The more you water and provide sunlight to a particular thought (by associating the thought with a particular emotion and actions), the more that thought grows into a full result.

This will be used to illuminate the seven levels of performance.

The Seven Levels of Performance

So what are the different types of mindset? There are seven levels of mindset Schneider has defined and validated through iPEC's work with thousands of individuals from all walks of life. Schneider has named these the seven levels of energy.[4] In this book, I interpret Schneider's seven levels of energy as the seven levels of performance.

These performance levels are characterized by core thought, core emotion, and core action. Each also corresponds to a particular energy level. The chart below summarizes my interpretation of iPEC's model for what I call the seven levels of performance:

PERFORMANCE LEVEL	CORE THOUGHT	CORE EMOTION	CORE ACTION	ENERGY LEVEL
L1: The Victim	Can't do anything	Sadness	Sluggish moves/plays	Catabolic
L2: The Aggressor	It's you or me	Anger	Angry moves/plays	Catabolic
L3: The Rationalizer	I/we did the best we could	Forgiveness	Moderate moves/plays	Mostly Anabolic
L4: The Servant	I want the best for the team/me	Altruism/gratitude	Team or self-moves/plays	Anabolic
L5: The Opportunist	I always see an opportunity	Curiosity; Peace, Confidence	New moves/plays	Anabolic
L6: The Strategist	I see 2-3 steps ahead of the move	Joy; Strong Confidence	Strategic moves/plays	Anabolic
L7: The Creator	I create any experience I want	Passion; Supreme Confidence	Creative moves/plays	Anabolic

Each performance level corresponds to one of two types of 'energy' or engagement identified by Schneider: catabolic and anabolic energy. Both energies are physiological states you experience every day.

Catabolic energy breaks down cells for quick bursts of energy and will raise stress hormones (such as cortisol) in the body. In the short-term, it serves the purpose of survival in certain situations (e.g. being attacked) through a fight-or-flight response; in the long-term, catabolic energy exhausts you. Anabolic energy, on the other hand, expands and heals the body through a release of hormones such as testosterone. It provides more of a long-term, growth-oriented state that serves sustainable success in all areas of life.[5]

LEVEL 1: THE VICTIM. This level of performance is all about having things happen *to you* and feeling as if you don't have any control over them (or even avoiding certain situations/people). The core thought is, *I can't do anything about this*. It triggers the emotion of apathy, which in turn triggers the core behavior of lethargy, lack of motivation, and avoidance. These are all characteristics of level one thinking, which can affect athletes, particularly after losses. The energy level is catabolic.

LEVEL 2: THE AGGRESSOR. The core thought is, *I win and you lose.* This triggers the emotion of anger because you're in a fight response now, which then triggers the behavior of conflict. It can be conflict with teammates, with an opposing team, with oneself, with a coach, or with time. Anything you view as a fight will result in level two. This is also very catabolic. Left unchecked, it can leave an incredible amount of cortisol in your system, which leads to stress and broken relationships.

You might be thinking to yourself, *Being aggressive is good. I perform well when I am aggressive.* True, you likely have had some really great performances when you were aggressive. However, if you take a step back, what you will see is that you were in a state of high alertness, which allowed you be at your best both offensively and defensively.

Further, the challenge with the aggressor mindset is that while you feel alert, it is difficult to repeat game after game. Moreover, it blocks you tapping into your creativity and intuition. Instead of the aggressor mindset, what you will learn about being in the zone is that there is an optimal level of alertness to have for your competitions and you can find this level at the higher mindsets (5 – 7) without the drawbacks of the aggressor mindset.

LEVEL 3: THE RATIONALIZER. This is all about tolerating, rationalizing, and coping with things. The core thought is, *Hey, I did my best. We did* *our best.* It's not about making excuses, it's trying to rationalize and cope with the result you're experiencing. This triggers somewhat of an emotion of forgiveness, which then triggers a resulting coping action (e.g. shrugging your shoulders). This level consists of some catabolic energy but begins to experience more anabolic energy.

LEVEL 4: THE SERVANT. This level is all about service and compassion. The core thought is about serving your team or your coach while having compassion toward yourself. The feelings triggered include compassion and gratitude. The core action triggered is one of service. This is anabolic in nature. It's strong, and it works really well in team sports. You always see the team captain, or sometimes the team servant, playing this role. The downside can be that if you're not careful to refuel yourself, you can get drained.

LEVEL 5: THE OPPORTUNIST. This level is all about seeing the opportunity in the situation. The core thought is, *I see the opportunity.* There's no longer a conflict going on. You will be able to turn anything into an opportunity, which will trigger an emotion of excitement and sometimes peace as well. The thought and emotion triggers an action oriented toward a new opportunity (e.g. in combat sports, spotting an opening in your opponent's movement and capitalizing on it). Level five provides a strong anabolic energy.

LEVEL 6: THE STRATEGIST. This mindset is about being able to see up to three moves ahead in the game. If you can sense the next three moves ahead, you will feel confident and certain. This is because you will tap into your creativity and intuition (more on the science behind this in the next chapter). The behavior triggered at this level is more like strategic plays, because you're attached to the big picture (e.g. as Wayne Gretzky would say about hockey plays—you know where the puck is going to be). It also has a strong focus in mastery. The core thought here is, *all experiences are valuable.* It's a little stronger than level five. The core emotions triggered are strong confidence, certainty, and joy because you know all experiences are making you a master, and there's a high level of trust involved. Level six provides powerful anabolic energy.

LEVEL 7: THE CREATOR. This is the penultimate of the zone. The core thought here is, *I believe anything is possible, and I can experience anything.* The emotion here is absolute passion, and the result is creation. Whereas level five was about seeing the opportunity in the situation and going after it, level six was about more of a strategic play. Level seven is about creating the strategic plays, not just being able to anticipate them. Because you're at such a high level of thinking and belief and tapping into your creativity and intuition, you're now making new moves and plays in your sport or taking high risks that you haven't taken before. Level seven provides the strongest level of anabolic energy possible.

These seven levels of performance formulate the backbone to much of my coaching with athletes and provide the foundation for helping athletes experience the zone more consistently. When I start working with an athlete, I have them take an assessment which measures their mindset across the seven levels of performance. It shows them where their dominant performance level is when the game/training is going well for them and when they come under stress in the game/training (stress meaning a trigger like fatigue, worry, anger over a referee call or opponent's foul). After our work together in several coaching sessions, I have the athlete re-take the assessment to gauge their progress.

Throughout this book, I also use these seven levels of performance to analyze performance-related challenges athletes experience and provide practical, step-by-step guide to overcoming these difficulties so zone-level performances will become a habit, not happenstance.

Key Points

- So much of peak performance is governing by the mind, but yet so few athletic programs and athletes spend enough resources in understanding and harnessing its power for their sport.
- The mind has two components: your brain and your consciousness, or

mindset.

- Mindset is the level of self-awareness you have of your true self.
- Focus has the power to determine your mindset; whatever you focus on, you will develop results in.
- Mindset is based on thoughts, which create emotions; emotions create actions; actions create results.
- The seven levels of performance provide a tool for understanding the mindset options available to you at any moment (the victim, the aggressor, the rationalizer, the servant, the opportunist, the strategist, and the creator).

chapter

2

The Zone

*"Nothing gives one person so much advantage over another
as to remain always cool and unruffled under all circumstances."*
THOMAS JEFFERSON

YOU'VE EXPERIENCED A GAME or a workout where time didn't seem to exist, things were effortless, and the result was simply one of the best performances you've had.

We all have had those times.

These experiences are called 'the zone' or 'being in the zone', and you will hold those times as pinnacles of your best experiences. And for a good reason: you work so hard, putting so much blood sweat and tears into getting to the top of your game. You might as well enjoy the fruits of your labor.

That is what this book is all about: making the zone experience a habit and not a happenstance. So, let us start with *what is the zone?*

The Zone as you Experience It

When you experience the zone, you have likely felt several of the following characteristics:

- Effortless and fluid
- Timelessness
- Little conscious thought
- Creativity
- Intuitive (you just 'knew' something was going to happen/your opponent would act a certain way before they did)

One of the main reasons you will experience these characteristics is because you will be immersed in the present with little conscious judgment made about the moment. In fact, when you're fully present, you will become so immersed in the experience itself that time will seem to slow down.

The Zone by Science

To more fully understand the zone state, let's turn to science for further explanations. There are two primary areas of human biology through which you can witness the zone state: the brain and the heart. The brain emits certain waves, depending on how active and alert it is for the activity you are performing. This chart summarizes four common brain states and their associated performance levels.

BRAIN STATE	PERFORMANCE STATE
DELTA BRAIN WAVES: 5 – 3hz	SLEEPING
THETA BRAIN WAVES: 3 – 8hz	LEARNING, MEDITATING
ALPHA BRAIN WAVES: 8 – 14hz	ZONE
BETA BRAIN WAVES: 14 – 35hz	HYPER ALERTNESS

Delta brain waves are associated with sleep patterns or deep meditation. Theta brain waves are associated with learning, integrating information, and meditation. Alpha Brain Waves are associated with the zone. Beta brain waves are associated with high alertness to the point of stress and anxiety. If you were to wear an EEG monitor on your head, you would be able to measure your brain waves and see these different waves.

When you are in the zone, your brain also emits five key neuro-chemical (messages transmitted in the brain) that are responsible for the amazing feelings you have. Steven Kotler, author of *The Rise of Superman,* lists these five:[6]

- **DOPAMINE:** the reward and motivation hormone for an exploratory act. It increases "attention, information flow, and pattern recognition in the brain and heart rate, blood pressure, and muscle firing timing in the body."
- **NOREPINEPHRINE:** the chemical that "increases arousal, attention, neural efficiency, and emotional control. In flow, it keeps us locked in target, holding distractions at bay."
- **ANANDAMIDE:** the chemical that "elevates mood, reduces pain, dilates blood vessels and bronchial tubes (adding respiration) and amplifies lateral thinking (our ability to link disparate ideas together)."

- **ENDORPHINS:** which "relieve pain and produce pleasure. The most common endorphin is one hundred times more powerful than medical morphine."
- **SEROTONIN:** provides the afterglow effect once the zone state is complete.

Kotler also shows that certain parts of your brain reduce their activity when in the zone. Most notably, parts of the prefrontal cortex, the part of the brain responsible for decision-making and cognitive thought, shut down temporarily. This state is called transient hypofrontality. This removes complexity from decision-making. In addition, other parts of the prefrontal cortex light up with other activity. This then produces several key benefits:[7]

- **Losing self-awareness:** losing your "introspective sense of self-awareness" (superior frontal gyrus quiets down)
- **Boosting creativity:** "creativity becomes freer flowing" (dorsolateral prefrontal cortex quiets down) and "creative self-expression increases" (medial prefrontal cortex becomes activated)
- **Increasing risk taking:** "risk taking becomes less frightening" (dorsolateral prefrontal cortex quiets down)
- **Maximizing strength:** we can "push our maximal strength closer to its absolute boundary" (due to the pain-killing neurochemicals being released)

In short, "with parts of the prefrontal cortex deactivated, there's no risk assessor, future predictor, or inner critic around to monitor the situation" which allows you to take risks, forget about pain, and dare new feats.[8]

A lot of mental performance training focuses on developing toughness—the grit you want to have to endure lots of pain and adversity. However, the benefit of the zone state is that your body takes care of the toughness for you through neurochemicals such as endorphins and anandamide. That is a good reason to become more efficient at getting in the zone.

Now for the heart. HeartMath® Institute has conducted over two decades of research on heart rate variability (the measurement of consistency in your heart rate). Through this research, HeartMath Institute found HRV is a powerful indicator of the physiological state called coherence: an optimal balancing and functioning of both your sympathetic nervous system (responsible for stress) and parasympathetic nervous system (responsible for calming). When both systems act together, you experience the right amount of 'alertness' for performance. It is my belief that the coherence state closely corresponds with the zone state and anabolic energy.

HeartMath Institute's chart below shows two different states (as measured by HRV): frustration or chaos, which is when the sympathetic nervous system is dominant; appreciation or coherence, which is when the sympathetic and parasympathetic nervous systems function optimally together.[9]

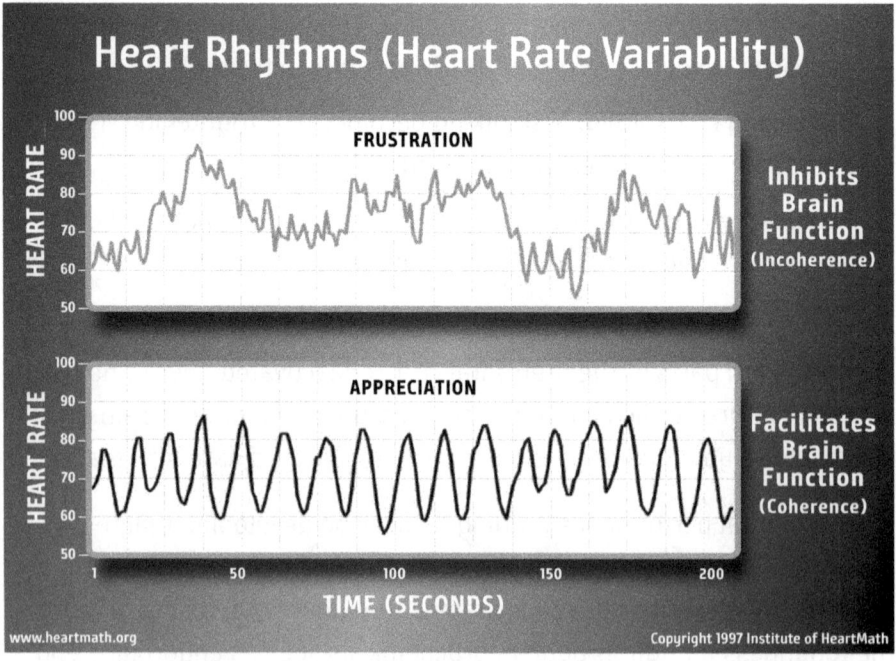

The key theme of brain and heart rate variability measures is this: the right level of alertness will be the zone state. On one extreme, you can have lower levels of alertness, which cause you to underperform (e.g. delta and theta brain waves). On the other extreme, there is hyper alertness would also cause you to underperform (e.g. beta brain waves or frustration). Finding the right level of alertness will create optimal performance. The inverted U graph shown below, first proposed by John Dodson and Robert Yerkes, demonstrates this concept:[10]

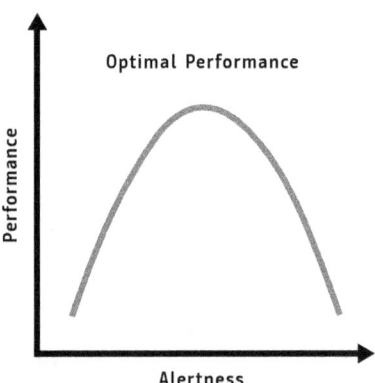

Conditions for Getting in the Zone

In his book, *Flow*, Mihaly Csikszentmihalyi researched thousands of athletes and professionals at the top of their game. He discovered several conditions that must be present for the zone state:[11]

- The activity is intrinsically rewarding (meaning you do it for the enjoyment of the sport)
- Clear goals and immediate feedback (knowing exactly what you are trying to accomplish and knowing if you are on target)
- Knowing that the task is doable; a balance between skill level and the challenge presented
- Total concentration and absorbed awareness (being immersed in what you are doing and being free of distractions)

To be in the zone, you need to find the activity enjoyable. This stimulates a sense of alertness for the activity. You also need to have a clear goal in mind of what you are looking to accomplish and have immediate feedback so you can stay on target. This provides your mind with the sense of clarity and certainty it needs for the zone state. You also need to have your skill set on par with the challenge. Lastly, you need to avoid distractions so you can be completely immersed in what you are doing.

The Zone Mindset

You may have been wondering: how does chapter one of this book, with its discussion of mindset via the seven levels of performance, relate to this chapter on the zone? I will conclude the chapter with an answer to this question.

The seven levels of performance describe all the performance options available to an athlete at any given moment. The levels that correspond to the zone state are as follows:

PERFORMANCE LEVEL	EMOTION(s)	ZONE STATE
LEVEL 4: The Servant	*Gratitude*	*The zone getaway. Beginning to access the zone will start here*
LEVEL 5: The Opportunist	*Curiosity; Peace; Confidence*	*The beginning stage of the zone*
LEVEL 6: The Strategist	*Joy; Strong Confidence*	*The mid-level stage of the zone*
LEVEL 7: The Creator	*Passion; Supreme Confidence*	*The highest stage of the zone*

LEVEL FOUR is the gateway to accessing the zone. Gratitude is the key gateway emotion for your state because it pulls you out of catabolic energy levels (levels 1-2) quickly. Moreover, as Tony Robbins says, "You can't be fearful and grateful at the same time."[12] Gratitude eliminates fear.

LEVEL FIVE is the beginning stage of the zone, as you will begin to see opportunities for the next play. As you spot the opportunities, you can capitalize on them in the moment. Curiosity, excitement, and peace are level five emotions.

LEVELS SIX AND SEVEN reach the mid-level and highest stages of the zone because you no longer need to 'try'; the game becomes effortless. You will become the game because you will be so engaged in the present moment. You will also be able to see moves one to two steps down the line, and you will start creating those sequences of moves yourself. Strong confidence, certainty, and passion are key emotions at these levels.

One caveat for these levels of performance is skill level: as mentioned about the conditions for the zone, having sufficient skill level for the challenge is necessary for these levels of performance. Once you have obtained sufficient skill level, then your mindset becomes of the utmost importance to put that skill to its most effective use. You can see my chapter on skill development for recommendations on speeding your skill development from a cognitive/mindset perspective as well.

An equal caveat to skill development: using all your skill depends on your mindset. As George Mumford, legendary mindfulness teacher and author of *The Mindful Athlete* says, "The real key to high performance and tapping into flow is the ability to direct and channel these strengths and skills fully in the present moment—and that starts in your mind."[13]

The remaining chapters will use the seven levels of performance and the conditions of getting in the zone to provide a handbook for getting in the zone, staying in the zone, and overcoming performance challenges such as loss and injury.

Key Points

- The zone is the place where your performance feels effortless, timeless, creative, intuitive, and amazing.
- The zone, scientifically, is when your brain in emitting alpha brain waves (8 – 14 hz) and your heart rate variability is in a coherent state.
- In the zone, your brain releases five neurochemicals that are responsible for the amazing feeling of the zone: dopamine (motivation), neuropronephrine (arousal), anandamide (pain reduction), endorphins (pain reduction), and serotonin (afterglow).
- In the zone, parts of your prefrontal cortex shut down and other parts light up, which allows you to: lose self-consciousness, be more creative and self-expressed, take more risks, and feel less pain.
- The seven levels of performance, levels 5 – 7 (the opportunist, the strategist, and the creator), correspond to the zone state.

chapter

3

~~~~~~~~~~~~~~~~~~

Getting in the Zone: The Mindset

"All things are ready if our minds be so."
HENRY V

THIS CHAPTER IS ALL ABOUT developing a process based on science and the seven levels of performance so that you can get into the zone more frequently. No two people are exactly the same. There might be some customization, some experimentation you have to do with this process, but in the end, regular practice will eventually get you there.

Common Approaches to Getting in the Zone

MISTAKE 1: No process. This mistake occurs when you show up with no plan for getting in the zone and leave it to happenstance. You can't just show up on the day of your event and hope for the best. That's not going to work.

MISTAKE 2: Thinking yourself into the zone. The reason why this won't work is because you're engaging the left part of your brain (logical reasoning), instead of the right side of your brain which is responsible for bodily connection, intuition, and creativity. The right side of your brain allows for access to your full potential.

MISTAKE 3: Using anger. You may try to use anger in an attempt at motivation. This is a level two (the aggressor) strategy that leads to a fight-or-flight response. It's a limited approach, and it's exhausting to do game after game, especially in a long string of games. You will try to boost your alertness, for sure, but you will end up over-amplifying your alertness. If you recall the alertness chart from chapter one, you will note that after a certain point, over-alertness negatively impacts performance (you are likely in a state of beta brainwaves and out of a coherent state, as measured by HRV).

MISTAKE 4: Trying to control the outcome. This is another common approach. You will focus so much on trying to win (well, that is what you *are* trying to do, isn't it?) that you will end up trying to control things you can't control (your opponents, the weather, a referee's call, the fans, etc.). This approach can inhibit the zone because it creates mind-body tension. The fact of the matter is this: you can't control your opponents, you can only control your responses to them. As the legendary Vale Tudo fighter and Brazilian Jiu-Jitsu master, Rickson Gracie, says, "You can't control the ocean, but you can learn to surf."[14]

Creating Your Zone Trigger

Some bad news: getting into the zone by habit is a process that requires practice. The good news is that you can take the guesswork out of it and once the process is ingrained, getting into the zone becomes a habit, not happenstance. In this section, I show you how to do this.

In his book, *The Art of Learning,* world champion chess master, and martial artist, Josh Waitzkin, recommends developing a 'trigger' that will get you into the zone state on a regular basis. "The point to this system of creating your own trigger is that a physiological connection is formed between the routine and the activity it precedes."[15] This sort of psycho-physiological (mind-body) connection is what will enable the triggering of the zone state in a short amount of time (once practiced enough).

Waitzken outlines a two-phase approach for developing your trigger. Phase one is to develop a four-to-five step process that will put your mind in that relaxed, but alert state.[16] I've laid out an outline of a five-step process based on the seven levels of performance which you can use and customize to meet your needs.

Phase two of Waitzken's approach involves gradually altering the process so as to make it both lower maintenance and more flexible so you can shorten it and use it in any situation.[17] When done so gradually, you will be able to enter into the zone state in a short amount of time in any environment.[18]

STEP ONE is to have clear, measurable goals that focus on the process. It is important to know what you're going to accomplish and be able to have that feedback as to whether you're on track or not. Having a clear and measurable goal provides you with the clarity and immediate feedback that Mihaly Csikszentmihalyi lists as an essential condition for getting into the zone.

Avoid outcome-based goals like 'to win the game.' That creates mind-body tension because you are trying to control something that's not in your absolute control. Remember, you can't control your opponent, you can only control yourself. One of the key conditions for getting in the zone is a sense of control. Therefore, you must focus on what you *can* control and let go of those things you cannot.

I recommend having three different goals for a game or big training event. When studying for my coaching certification with iPEC, our CORE performance dynamics training discussed three types of important goals athletes can set for their performance.

The first, your A-goal, is the ideal scenario. It may be to flawlessly execute your game plan. Alternatively, it may be to score a certain amount of points or hit a certain pace during the race, depending on your sport. For instance, a basketball player may want to sink ninety-five percent of the three-pointers shot, or an MMA fighter may want to land ninety-five percent of all significant strikes. Nonetheless, your ideal goal should remain within your grasp and not be focused just on winning (but would contribute to winning in a big way).

The B-goal is the backup plan when it becomes clear you can't achieve plan A. This may be a backup game plan or it may be moves that are more manageable for you to accomplish. For instance, a basketball player might decide to move around more on the court, set more picks, or have more assists. The MMA fighter may want to focus on executing their backup game plan.

The C-goal is a scenario that you know you can achieve no matter what. You likely would make this goal one of simply having fun and learning. One of the best anecdotes for nearly professional athletes who freeze up under pressure is to have fun.

Having three different goals is similar to diversifying your investment portfolio. Even if you don't meet your A- or B-goal, you can always reach your C-goal. Therefore, you will never have to worry about being frustrated that you didn't meet your goals—everyone can always have fun and learn.

Even if it is half-time, between a round in a fight, or halfway through a race, you can remind yourself that you can have fun and learn even if the A- or B-goals are not within your reach. That will be a boost to your mindset because it keeps you in control.

David Rock, author of *Your Brain at Work,* shows the brain science behind this sort of approach to multiple goals. When your brain has unmet expectations via unmet goals, you will experience a drop in dopamine levels (the motivation hormone) and a 'threat response' (which will trigger a victim or aggressor mindset).[19] Hence the deflated feeling you have when something isn't meeting your expected goal. If you only have one goal, like winning, you can trigger this loss of dopamine when it seems you may not win, which means losing the zone state and making it more difficult to access your creativity and intuition when you need it most.

However, if you can exceed the expectations you set for yourself, there will be an increase in dopamine levels in your brain and a 'reward' feeling for things that go better than planned.[20] This will give you a mental edge in the game, an extra boost of motivation, and positive feelings you can use to fuel improved performance. By having a few different goals, one of which you can achieve no matter what (the C-goal), it becomes a lot easier to exceed expectation and thus keep your dopamine levels high.

STEP TWO is gratitude. This is a level four (the servant) strategy that involves fostering a sense of gratitude for the ability to play the sport, the ability to compete, your teammates, the skills you've developed, and your coaches.

Gratitude is important because it cannot co-exist with fear. If you put yourself in a state of complete gratitude, you will eliminate fear. Fear is one of the biggest detractors to remaining in the zone. When you're fearful, you're not going to be able to access your full potential. Your ability to take risks will be limited. This leads to the fight or flight response, which as we've said before, is detrimental to performance.

Before your game or event, write down three things you're grateful for. They can be related to the event or life in general. Then breathe those three things into your heart. Take a deep breath through your nose, imagine the air going into your heart, pulling all that you're grateful for into your heart, and breathe out. It will only take two minutes of this type of 'gratitude breathing' for your brain and heart to sync.[21] This step is your zone gateway: gratitude is the gateway emotion.

STEP THREE is to have fun. This is a level five (the opportunist) strategy. Once you've set your goals and practiced gratitude, it's time to put a smile on your face and focus on having fun. Remember when you first fell in love with the game? Bring that memory back into the current performance. This approach is essentially putting your C-goal into practice.

Following this strategy will lead to a huge energy boost. It relieves pressure and will get you into a level five state, because it will be so much easier to see the opportunities before you, and you will be able to capitalize on each opportunity. When you focus on fun it becomes easier to tap into your creativity as the pressure will be off and some looseness will be allowed into your mind and body (not too loose, just the right level of relaxed alertness).

STEP FOUR is to love the experience. This step is a level six (the strategist) strategy. The finishing touches involve focusing on enjoying the experience. Fall in love with the sounds and smells of your sport. If you start to fall in love with the experience itself, then you will shift to a higher state, level six.

This is an incredibly powerful state that allows you to be in the zone. You will forget about judgment and criticism. You will be able to tap into your creativity and intuition without having to think about it. That, in turn, means that much more of your skill is available to use in the moment.

This is where you experience timelessness, effortlessness, creativity, and an overall amazing feeling.

> ZONE TIP
>
> *It is important to have clear, undistracted focus once the game begins. Distractions will take you out of the zone immediately. Developing your focus—that ability to keep your focus on the present moment and the task at hand—will directly contribute to your ability to get into the zone and stay in the zone.*

This four-step process will require some practice before getting in the zone becomes automatic. However, it will provide immediate benefits, even just going through steps one and two. When you experiment with this process and make tweaks for what works and doesn't, you will find your own version of a flawless formula that gets you into the zone each time.

When I work with athletes and teams, I help them customize this formula and practice it relentlessly so it becomes a habit.

ZONE TRIGGER SUMMARY:

- Step 1: create ABC goals
- Step 2: practice gratitude
- Step 3: focus on fun and learning
- Step 4: fall in love with the experience

Increasing Intuition

One of the characteristics of getting the zone is your heightened ability to tap into your intuition (your gut feeling of just 'knowing' something). Your intuition is a powerful source of information for athletic performance because it can give you a heads-up as to what your opponent is going to do before they even do it. It may give you a sense that you should use a particular technique for a particular environment.

In addition to developing and practicing your zone trigger, you can practice increasing your intuition. Commander Mark Devine shows three practices for increasing your sense of intuition in his book, *The Way of the Seal*. Being a navy seal, a martial artist, and having researched practices from several warrior traditions and modern psychology, Commander Devine has compiled some outstanding practical advice for increasing your intuition.

1. Combine focused and relaxed awareness. When you practice focused awareness, you look intently through your eyes to pick up every detail, using them like laser beams. "When you use your eyes in this way, your conscious mind is fully engaged in observing and processing information."[22] When you practice relaxed awareness, you "defocus your eyes, allowing information to flow through the eyes and into the mind as if they were windows." This allows information to be imprinted into your subconscious mind and be available for use later. The key to tapping "into your intuition is to shift between focused and relaxed awareness"[23] depending on the situation. For moments that are more relaxed in intensity during a game or practice, use relaxed awareness to gather all the information about the environment and opponents. For moments of more focused performance, use focused awareness to heighten your shots, strikes, attacks, plays, etc. (depending on your sport).

2. Increase sensory perception. Your five senses provide a lot of valuable information you can use to gauge the situation, your opponents, your team, and your coaches. This information feeds into your intuition, which will help you to make split-second decisions about the next move or play. To develop your senses, practice sensory deprivation for several of the five senses[24]:

    - Sight: Close your eyes for up to a minute. Notice what you see when you close them. Now, open your eyes. Notice what you see, especially when you look more intently. Write down any observations.

    - Sound: Cup your hands around your ears for up to a minute. Notice what you hear. Now, take your hands off your ears. Notice what you hear. Write down any observations.

- Smell: Pinch your nose shut for up to a minute (breathe through your mouth). Notice if you can or cannot smell anything. Now, take your hand off your nose and breathe through your nose. Notice what you smell. Write down any observations.

You can combine these exercises. For instance, you can close your eyes and cup your ears and follow the same pattern. The point is that deprivation, then return of your senses will sharpen your awareness of the information being received by that sense.

3. Uncover hidden beliefs. You and I have beliefs that have become subtly ingrained in our subconscious mind from our life experiences. These beliefs are not necessarily good or bad, right or wrong; however, "some of these beliefs may cause your subconscious mind to work against our conscious desires in direct and indirect ways."[25] For instance, they may cause you to become outraged over a referee call you disagree with during a championship game; they may make you adverse to stringent, methodical practice. In any event, there may be beliefs that are holding you back and preventing you from accessing your intuition. To identify these beliefs, look for situations that trigger you and elicit catabolic emotions like anger, worry, doubt, and lethargy. These emotions indicate a hidden belief is at work. To removing these hidden beliefs, you can use the affirmations found in the morning power ritual in chapter eight to replace the old beliefs with new ones. Ultimately, however, you may need to seek the help of a coach to do the necessary inner work to replace these outdated beliefs with ones that serve you.

Key Points

- Common mistakes for getting in the zone include not having a process, trying to think yourself into the zone, anger-based techniques, and focusing on the outcome.

- Getting into the zone is more easily facilitated by creating a zone trigger, which is a process that eventually trains your mind and body for getting in the zone on command.
- The zone trigger you develop can involve setting proper goals which provide the clarity of purpose and allow you to get immediate feedback as to whether you are on track or not. Using a three-fold set of goals that are within your control will facilitate this process (these include strategic, process, and fun and learning goals).
- The zone trigger can involve practicing gratitude before your competition, which will help eliminate fear and set you up to begin entering into the zone state.
- The zone trigger can include a focus on fun and learning (one of your goals) which will make it easier to spot opportunities opening up in the competition.
- The zone trigger can also include a focus on loving the experience of competition itself, which will allow you to develop a strategic mindset.
- Your intuition supplies you with valuable 'hunches' that can allow you to make powerful, split-second decisions that fuel peak performance. You can develop your intuition through exercises such as relaxed/focused awareness, sensory deprivation, and uncovering hidden beliefs.

chapter

4

Getting in the Zone: Skill Development

"Excellence is a habit."
ARISTOTLE

AS MENTIONED IN THE previous two chapters, the other key fundamentals to getting into the zone are having the right balance between skill level and the challenge that you're undergoing. If the challenge is too big for your skill set, it's going to be difficult to get in the zone. In addition, if your skill set's bigger than the challenge, it's going to be difficult to get in the zone (since you will be too bored to have enough alertness). Having a good balance between the two really produces that zone state.

Proper skill development and conditioning requires a great skills coach to help you develop the right technique, form, exercises, and repetitions for your sport. Both skill development and conditioning result from the quality and quantity of repetition with the proper adjustments made for the timing of the season and your body. For most of your athletic experiences, this likely forms the heart of your training.

While much of skill development takes place with repetition and feedback from your skills and conditioning coaches, quite a bit is governed by your mindset. The beliefs and the state of your mind will drastically affect both the effectiveness and speed at which your skill and conditioning levels develop.

I want to show you how mindset affects your rate of skill development and provide a process you can use for developing the right mindset for training.

Skill Development: From the Seven Levels of Performance

The seven levels of performance don't just describe the mindset options for the game, they also describe the mindset options available for training. Once you become more aware of the dominant mindset you approached training with in the past, you can start consciously choosing which mindset(s) you'd like to approach training with so you get the most value out of your sessions in the future.

LEVEL 1: The victim. At this level, skill development just happens to you, there's nothing you can do about it, either it's going to happen or it's not. There will be a low level of motivation, a low level of belief in oneself, and low level of desire and energy and effort put forward to acquire and own the skills.

You might experience this level when first learning a new move or after failing to nail a move after countless hours of practice. You might say to yourself, *Nothing I do works.* You might give up trying to acquire the skill or avoid trying it in order to save yourself the embarrassment of failure.

In either circumstance, this is a victim mindset that drastically inhibits your mind from being open to learning the skill and building the proper neural networks required for making the skill second nature.

LEVEL 2: The aggressor. This is a level in which you will believe you need to fight against yourself, fight against time, or fight against someone/something else in order to acquire skills. At this level, your motivation to learn the skill grows. You will put a lot of effort in your practices at this level.

In the short-run, the aggressor can create a powerful burst of energy that may be needed to push yourself past your limits during the last stages of an intense strength and conditioning workout. It also may serve you well to push yourself in final minutes of an intense skill workout, team skirmish or sparring match. For an intentional and short duration, the aggressor mindset can serve you.

While the aggressor state is powerful in the short-run, there are long-term drawbacks. The aggressor mindset produces mind/body tension. Even though you will experience a quick burst of energy, it will hold back your long-term potential: it closes off access to your creativity and intuition, which is important in developing the 'feel' of a move and your body.

LEVEL 3: The rationalizer. Skill development and conditioning at this level is all about doing the best you can. At this level, your mind will believe that you have certain limitations for the given training session and that achieving the particular goal likely won't happen, but you will try your best. Alternatively, after a training session that didn't go so well, your mind will cope with the results by reassuring yourself that you did the best you could.

The benefit of this mindset is that it allows you to move past a victim or aggressor reaction to a training session that didn't go well. For instance, if you have been trying to nail a move in practice for you can't remember how long and you still can't nail it, you might experience a victim or aggressor reaction. Staying at one or two of these levels too long can be detrimental to your growth. Therefore, when you find yourself coping with your setback, and saying that you did the best you could, you are moving past the victim or aggressor mindset, which helps you move into anabolic energy.

The drawback to this mindset is that it still limits your growth if you hang around it too long. You will never dare to believe and trust that you can nail a new move or achieve a new level of conditioning. If all you keep telling yourself is, "I'll try it again," then you may never achieve success. As Yoda, in Star Wars V, says, "Do or do not; there is no try."[26]

LEVEL 4: The servant. With this mindset, skill development and conditioning will be about your team: your motivation will be to help your teammates and develop techniques and plays that benefit them and the team as a whole. During intense workouts, you motivate yourself to get through the workout by motivating the team as a whole to push to new levels.

The benefit of this mindset for skills and conditioning is that it begins to take you outside yourself by providing a powerful reason for improvement: others. The shared camaraderie in any team sport is a powerful motivator. When everyone pushes each member of the team to improve, your performance can only go up.

The drawback to this mindset is that if you remain there too long, or make it your sole mindset for practice, then you can become drained energetically. The reason for the drain is that you may end up neglecting your own legitimate needs in service of the team. Moreover, you may even miss seeing opportunities for your own development (e.g. refinements in technique) due to having a complete team focus.

LEVEL 5: The opportunist. This mindset will provide a sweet spot for skill development and conditioning. This is because you will be able to see an opportunity in everything. At this level, you will cease to see 'mistakes' and instead see opportunities to get better. At this mindset, you won't be able to make lemonade out of lemons (that is a coping mindset, which is level three), but you will be able to see all sorts of new opportunities available with that lemon. That means training sessions that don't go as planned provide you with enormous learning value for improvement.

The benefit of this mindset is that skill development and conditioning grow exponentially since you're open to the trial and error of learning. It will keep you energized and motivated. Having that enthusiasm for development will allow you to acquire the skill faster since it prevents you from closing down your mind with judgment and opens you to correcting a move or technique more efficiently. Because you can learn the proper technique, this allows your neural pathways to develop the proper connections so that the move or technique becomes second nature. Furthermore, practice at the level five stage is much more fun! Judgment about 'wrong' moves or 'mistakes' significantly lessens, and you will be able to feel peaceful and excited about the opportunities presented to you in learning. As the two head instructors (Rener and Ririon Gracie) of the famous Gracie Academy in Los Angeles, CA say, "Keep it playful."[27]

The drawback of this mindset is that you can become distracted with so many opportunities for development. That might take the form of getting excited by the latest and greatest training technique, diet, etc. and not sticking with a good plan you started at the beginning of the season. To be clear, gaining the edge through a cutting-edge approach is not a bad thing; however, changing the plan up simply because you are excited by a new opportunity may or may not serve your development in the long run. Prioritizing opportunities and aligning them with principles of consistency and focus will help keep your enthusiasm in check.

LEVEL 6: The strategist. This mindset builds off level five and becomes even stronger since your view of skill development and conditioning becomes about the love of the experience. Loving the experience itself gives you a strategist mindset as you will come to realize every experience in training, competition, and life has value. This mindset produces joy because you will know that every experience in life and your sport has value, no matter what. Setbacks, losses, and 'bad practices' can still induce joy because they not only provide learning, but they are a part of the big picture of life.

The benefit of this mindset is that you not only improve your rate of skill development, as in level five, but your enjoyment of the process skyrockets. You will be connected to the bigger picture and you will be able to become a more strategic and patient athlete in your training. You will also be vastly more creative at this mindset, since you can tap into your creativity and intuition due to the low level of judgment you will place on your training experiences.

The drawback of this mindset is that some people may not be able to relate to your elevated mindset. Your teammates may not share your sense of joy over a practice or game that didn't go their way. While you will be convinced of the sense that you are always winning and getting better, others may not be able to see that big picture of mastery so easily. So be cautious to meet people where they are at after something that did not go their way. Beyond this drawback, there isn't much else detracting from the strategist mindset for an athlete. It is a place of deep joy, high intuition and creativity, and deep belief you can make things happen.

LEVEL 7: The creator. This mindset is the penultimate in terms of its ability to make any experience you desire happen as fast as possible. That means training will be about creating the experiences you desire. If you desire to nail a particular move and feel great about it, then at this mindset you will be able to do it. At this level, you live Yoda's advice: "Do."

The benefit of this mindset is the ability to master any skill level faster and at a higher level of quality than you would have believed possible under any other mindset. Moreover, your quality of this experience will be effortless and naturally feels amazing. Your creativity and intuition will be at the highest level, since you will have no judgment of your experience.

The drawback to this level is that it can be a difficult mindset to sustain for a long period of time due to its intensity and the natural difficulty of not placing judgments on your experience for long periods. Other than this drawback, the creator mindset has its place when you are already at a high-level mindset (levels five through six) and wish to take it up a notch to nail a move or workout.

As you can see, each level of performance has a benefit and drawback. The key to understanding and using the seven levels of performance is to understand which situation and level will serve you best. Given the nature of skill development, I recommend a level five (the opportunist) mindset for nearly all of your practices. It doesn't take too much to shift into this mindset, whereas levels six and seven may require more time and intensive work (depending on the person). For that reason, level five is much more repeatable over time for your practices and will also provide you with a consistent level of fun.

Putting the Seven Levels of Performance to Work

As I recommended in the previous chapter, with developing a 'trigger' you can use for getting in the zone, I would also recommend one to use when preparing for your practices. Again, you don't want to leave things to happenstance. It isn't a matter of practice makes perfect, rather, perfect practice makes perfect. In other words, showing up to practice with the right mindset allows you to get the most out of your hard work.

I will outline a recommended routine you can use to develop your 'training trigger' so that level five becomes a regular experience. Just as in the previous chapter, a two-phased approach still applies for generating the trigger. First, create the process and practice it regularly. Second, shorten the process over time so that within just a few minutes (or perhaps even seconds!) you can trigger your opportunist mindset.

STEP 1: Gratitude. This is a level four (the servant) strategy that involves fostering a sense of gratitude for the ability to participate in your sport and practice it. Some people, through no fault of their own, cannot enjoy the level of physical freedom and skill you and I can in our sports. Sometimes you and I can take it for granted what we can do. Therefore, fostering gratitude for your training is powerful.

As I mentioned in the previous chapter, gratitude is important because it cannot co-exist with fear. If you put yourself in a state of complete gratitude, you will eliminate the fear, annoyance, coping, and other inhibitors to higher levels of performance. It is also relatively simple to put yourself into a grateful state.

Before your practice, think of one to three things you are grateful for. Then breathe those things into your heart. Take a deep breath through your nose, imagine the air going into your heart, pulling all that you're grateful for into your heart, then breathe out.

STEP 2: Learning and fun. This is a level five (the opportunist) strategy. Ask yourself what you would like to focus on learning (you may want to consult with your coach). It may be correcting a move or re-enforcing an existing one. Establish a clear and certain mental picture of what it looks like to have achieved this learning goal. Breathe into this achievement, feeling the clarity and certainty of the accomplishment.

Next, bring to mind a time when you had a lot of fun at practice or somewhere else in your life. Focus on what made the event so much fun and breathe in that experience. Chances are the experience will put a smile on your face as you remember it. Keeping that smile, ask yourself one thing you can do during practice to inject some fun into it. It may be smiling, laughing, telling jokes, or doing something completely spontaneous.

At first, both of these steps may take between five to ten minutes as you practice them. Gradually over time, as you modify them, it may only take thirty seconds to achieve the same effect.

As you seek to customize these steps for your own benefit, feel free to add these steps to any other steps you take to prep for practice. You may already have a nutritional, stretching, and meditative-based approach to prepping for your training sessions. Feel free to be creative in mixing in these two steps; they marry well with almost any pre-training prep.

Skill Development Strategy: Deep Practice

Daniel Coyle, author of *The Talent Code* outlines the latest research into skill development, both from a biological perspective as well as from a training perspective.

From a biological viewpoint, the key finding of Coyle's research is that the key to elite skill is myelination of nerve fibers in the brain. Myelin is the fatty insulation that protects nerve fibers in the brain. While nerve fibers and synapses were thought to be the most important factor in skill development, scientists are now learning that the degree of myelination over the nerve fibers is also essential. "It determines and increases signal strength, speed, and accuracy."[28] Coyle goes so far as to say that "skill is myelin insulation that wraps neural circuits and that grows according to certain signals."[29]

From a training perspective, Coyle finds that the best strategy to improve myelin insulation is what he calls 'deep practice.' Deep practice is a particular way of training that forces you to correct mistakes on the spot. By "struggling in certain targeted ways—operating at the edges of your ability, where you make mistakes—makes you smarter."[30]

Coyle outlines the three rules of deep practice that will guide your deep practice training.[31]

Chunk it up. This is an intuitive principle that you have likely used at some point in your athletic career. It involves seeing the whole picture of the activity (a technique, the game plan, etc.), dividing the entire activity into its smallest parts, and slowing down and speeding up the practice of each part to learn every component.

Repeat it. Once you have broken down the key parts of the activity, then repeat, repeat, repeat. However, with deep practice, you don't need to overdo it. "Spending time is more effective—but only if you are still at the sweet spot at the edge of your capabilities, attentively building and honing your circuits."[32]

Feel it. Feeling every aspect of the activity is important for deep practice. It allows you to become absorbed in the entire process so you develop an intuitive understanding of the activity and can immediately feel a mistake that needs to be corrected.

To apply the deep practice strategy to your training, work with your coaches to identify specific training practices that will force you to fail quickly and correct those mistakes in the moment. Since most training is broken down into chunks by your coaches, spend more time practicing at the edge of your ability and feeling the entire activity so you can immediately sense any mistake that should be corrected. Deep practice is about picking a target, striving for it, and evaluating the gap between the target and your effort.[33] To support you in this strategy, adopt the level five mindset (the opportunist) so that mistakes don't embarrass you or trigger frustration. Instead, mistakes will be seen as genuine learning opportunities that you can be excited about and will serve to maintain your confidence.

When you combine this strategy with the insights from Anders Ericcson's research on the 10,000-hour theory (that 10,000 hours of practice is required for mastery), you get a simple formula Coyle puts forward to guide your training: "Deep practice x 10,000 hours = world-class skill."[34]

Key Points

- Having the proper skill and conditioning for your competitions is important for you to be able to get into the zone.
- Mindset plays a major role in your rate of improvement in training; the seven levels of performance will give you seven options from which to approach your training sessions.

- The recommended mindset is level five (the opportunist) as this will help you quickly spot new learning and keep your mindset playful as you train.

- Developing your 'training trigger' to use before practice can help you enter into the level five mindset much quicker so you can get the most out of your practices.

- Deep practice is a skill development strategy that maximizes myelin insulation (key to skill development) by forcing you to make mistakes and correct them quickly; work with your coach to identify ways to fail and learn movements quickly.

PART II

STAYING IN THE ZONE

The first part of this book was about equipping you with the information you need to start getting in the zone on a more regular basis. You learned about the Seven Levels of Performance, scientific qualities of the zone, building a Zone Trigger, and building a Training Trigger.

The second part of the book is about some of the things that can get in the way of you getting in the zone. These are challenges that athletes face in any sport and you will see some practical steps for how to overcome these challenges. I call these challenges "Zone Inhibitors". There are more inhibitors that could be discussed, but these are some of the common challenges you likely may face as an athlete.

chapter 5

Zone Inhibitor: Fear and Worry

"The only thing we have to fear is fear itself."
U.S. PRESIDENT FRANKLIN D. ROOSEVELT

FEAR AND WORRY CAN MAKE you do funny things. You can be the most accomplished, well-trained athlete and yet choke because of fear. You can be the most talented player, but if paralyzed by fear, you will make the wrong move at the wrong time. Alternatively, you won't use all of your potential: you will play a reserved game, holding back just to make sure the thing you fear most won't come to fruition.

Fear and worry are catabolic emotions (the victim and aggressor mindsets). These emotions can serve a certain purpose like alerting you to a life-threatening situation. However, for athletic performance, these emotions will drain your energy reserves and block your ability to tap into your creativity and intuition. Biologically, when you experience fear and worry your sympathetic nervous system kicks into high gear, releasing all sorts of stress hormones into your body (such as cortisol). This is your body's safety mechanism to protect yourself from primal life and death dangers (together with the parasympathetic nervous system, it comprises the autonomic nervous system). They will make accessing the opportunist, and any stronger mindset, where you enter the zone difficult.

If you are a professional athlete, performance drops can have big impacts: reduced monetary payout, increased pressure to perform at the next event (and fear of what happens if you don't), less enjoyment of the sport itself, and over time, being fired.

If you are an amateur athlete, this could mean anything from not making the professional team to not making your personal bests (no small gripe when you sacrifice your spare time with friends, family, and comfort to train for your event).

Causes of Fear and Worry

Fear and worry exist when you think of a future scenario you don't want to experience. When you let your mind drift to future scenarios, you engaging in horizontal thinking (allowing your awareness to drift to the past or future scenarios). Engaging in horizontal thinking (visualization exercises are an exception) can open the doors to fear and worry because you can't control the future moments and this can open the opportunity for the ego to start playing tricks on you.

The most common future scenario athletes entertain is the 'what if' scenario. "What if I try this move and we lose the game because it doesn't work out? What if I go out too aggressively in the first part of the race and run out of gas?" You may not be fully aware of these thought or try to fight them off. Chances are, you have experienced the 'what if' scenarios before high-pressure games and intense workouts.

I don't mean to sound dismissive of the 'what ifs' of life. There is an appropriate time to consider implications of future decisions. Engaging in smart and prudent decision-making is necessary, and that process does involve considering future scenarios that result from your decisions (what if). Therefore, there will be times you need to engage in a sort of horizontal thinking when engaging in planning and decision-making for important areas of your life and sport.

However, when preparing for your game or competition, especially the day(s) leading up to it, it is important to be aware of how easily the mind can engage in horizontal thinking, as this can allow fear and worry to seep into your mindset.

Moreover, during competition, you may have experienced yourself dwelling on the mistake you made a few minutes ago (whether it was a missed shot in a game, going out too hard at the beginning of a race, or being taken down in a fight). This worry can take you out of the present moment and divided your awareness. This state means that you will be less effective at controlling your actions in the present moment and tapping into your creativity and intuition. You may miss the next opportunity presented to you, causing yet another item to tack onto your worry list. This process can become a vicious cycle if you are not able to break back into the present moment.

"Overcoming Fear and Worry": The Conventional Wisdom

When it comes to strategies and tactics for handling fear and worry, most conventional wisdom boils down to this approach: be courageous and 'overcome' fear. Since fear is natural to the human experience (and it is), you will likely exercise some intestinal fortitude and take action in the face of your fear. You will come up with all sorts of ways to fight fear, manage fear, overcome fear . . . you name it, it's been researched, advocated, and used.

Here is what is missing in the conventional wisdom: 'fighting' fear requires energy. Fighting the fear you experience inside creates division within yourself. You have pitted yourself against yourself. Internal division wastes energy and will prevent you from accessing all your skills. Face it: while your energy stores are renewable, they can be depleted because you only have so much at any time. Not just physical energy, but emotional and mental energy. If you spend energy 'fighting' fear, then you are wasting energy you could be putting into the performance at hand.

Contrary to conventional wisdom, I do not believe the only way to move past fear is to 'overcome' fear. There is another alternative. One far more powerful, but it requires practice.

Fearlessness and Worry-Free

Instead of overcoming fear and worry, why not be without fear and worry in the first place? Stop trying to overcome fear and worry. Practice fearlessness and be worry-free. You won't have to create internal division within you. Instead, you will have a holistic integration of all of your abilities. If you are fearless, you will have much more energy you can put into the performance at hand.

Not only that, but you will also have a huge advantage over your competitor: you will have much greater access to creativity and intuition. Being able to use your creativity and intuition to respond in the moment will allow you pull off moves, make plays, and endure pain in ways that make spectators and commentators scratch their heads in awe.

Fear and worry do not exist when you are fully engaged in the present moment. All you have in the present moment are situations: circumstances you can handle because you can take action in the present moment. When you become fully alive and passionate about the present moment, you will put yourself in a fearless state. You will be in the zone.

Putting Fearlessness to Work

Fear and worry are emotions triggered by a stimulus. The stimulus may have been drifting into horizontal thinking, or it may have been making a mistake mid-way through the competition. Either way, that stimulus has now created a response that is registered as fear or worry. The key in this formula is that there was a stimulus (e.g. horizontal thinking) and a response (e.g. fear).

To be fearless and worry-free you need to create a space between the stimulus and response. George Mumford, mindfulness teacher and author of *The Mindful Athlete,* says that the center space "between stimulus and response is like the eye of the hurricane."[35] The eye of the hurricane for you is the calm but alert focus that characterizes optimal performance (the zone).

Creating this center space is a return to the present moment where fear and worry cannot exist. However, it also means more than just returning to the present moment. It means being in the present moment with a specific mindset that has transcended fear and worry, a mindset that does not involve fighting or coping with fear and worry.

Since fear and worry trigger the sympathetic nervous system into action, you will need a counterbalance to these stress hormones: the parasympathetic nervous system. If the sympathetic nervous system creates stress hormones, the sympathetic nervous system generates relaxation and triggers the release of relaxation hormones such as acetylcholine. As Mumford says, "the sympathetic nervous system is the accelerator, pressing the pedal to the metal . . . and the parasympathetic nervous system puts on the breaks and slows everything down."[36] Being fearless and worry-free, especially if you are experiencing a stimulus and response event around fear and worry, means engaging your parasympathetic nervous system in this 'center space,' this 'eye of the hurricane.'

The process I recommend for returning to fearlessness and a state of being worry-free not only engages the parasympathetic nervous system to put the brakes on the sympathetic nervous system, but it actually places both systems in optimal sync.

Seal Commander Mark Devine, who I referred to in chapter three on developing your intuition, provides a helpful practice for transforming catabolic emotions into anabolic emotions. His tool is called DIRECT: "detect, interdict, redirect, energize, communicate, and train."[37] You can practice this tool anytime you sense a catabolic emotion like fear or worry. I've combined his DIRECT tool with the seven levels of performance and the HeartMath breathing technique for maximum effect.

> **STEP 1:** Acceptance. You will need to foster an attitude of acceptance around the emotion. Allow yourself to fully feel the emotion in your body and accept it as it is. Notice how it affects your muscles, heart rate, and other sensations in your body.[38]
>
> **STEP 2:** Create space. Once you have accepted the emotion, create space between it.[39] Breathe deep using the HeartMath breathing technique (it brings your sympathetic and parasympathetic nervous systems into optimal sync).[40]
>
> - Breathe through your nose (for four to five seconds) and imagine you are bringing that breath directly into your heart.
> - Now exhale (for four to five seconds) out of your mouth, imagining your breathe leaving your heart area.
> - Continue this pattern for up to two minutes.
>
> **STEP 3:** DIRECT to a healthy (anabolic) emotion.[41] For this practice, you will focus on gratitude. This is the gateway emotion that will allow you to shift back into the higher mindsets such as levels five through seven.
>
> - As you breathe into your heart, bring to mind something you are grateful for in your life. Specifically, bring this object of gratitude into your heart and feel the gratitude there.

- Continue this breathing pattern and bring to your heart as many items of gratitude as you need. You can return to an optimal state in a concise period of time following this pattern. To lock your body in this state for a longer period, spend ten to fifteen minutes following this pattern.

ZONE TIP
You can also place your hands over your heart to bring further stimulation to your heart and the entire experience.

This process can be performed anytime you notice yourself experiencing fear and worry: perhaps the night before a competition, during half-time, before the walk-out, or while stretching during warm-ups before the competition. This process will shift your emotions out of fear and worry. Remember, as Tony Robbins says, you can't be fearful and grateful at the same time.[42]

Once you have achieved a fearless and worry-free state, you can further boost your mindset to the opportunist or strategist mindset more easily. I recommend following steps three and four of your zone trigger (fun, and loving the experience) to boost your mindset up to these levels.

Key Points

- Fear and worry are catabolic emotions that will inhibit your performance and prevent you from getting into the zone.
- Fear and worry are caused by horizontal thinking, which takes you out of the present moment and into the past or future.
- Most people think they need to overcome fear and worry through courage. A better way is to be fearless and worry-free.
- You can practice fearlessness by first practicing the DIRECT tool, combined with gratitude and the HeartMath breathing technique.

chapter

6

~~~~~~~~~~~~~~~~

Zone Inhibitor: Loss

"It is not the critic who counts...the credit belongs to the man...who strives valiantly."
U.S. PRESIDENT THEODORE ROOSEVELT

UNLESS YOU ARE SUPERMAN, at some point you are going to face a loss (even Superman had his struggles with kryptonite). You know what can happen to your mindset when you lose (or don't meet your ultimate goal), right?

You might doubt your ability, or you may feel like there wasn't anything you could have done (level one, victim mindset). You may get frustrated and angry (level two, aggressor mindset). You might try to brush it off as an anomaly and tell yourself you did the best you could, given the circumstances (level three, rationalizer mindset).

All of these reactions to loss or underperformance are normal. Ultimately, it would be nice to skip these reactions and keep your mindset high, at say the level five, opportunist level. After much practice, perhaps with the help of a coach, you will be able to do so as a habit with little effort. However, until you reach this state, you will want to create a process to follow to 'trigger' yourself into a higher mindset.

Just as with the zone and practice triggers you created in chapters three and four, you will want to have a trigger to bounce quickly back from a loss or underperformance. In the section below, I outline a process that is based on the seven levels of performance that you can customize for your sport.

The Process

STEP 1: Cope with the loss (the rationalizer). As a first step to regaining your mindset, I recommend seeing the loss in perspective. To do this, you are going to create a 'loss scale.'

On a sheet of paper, draw a vertical scale. On the bottom of the scale write a one, in the middle of the scale write a fifty, and at the top of the scale write one hundred. This is the scale you will use to assess the level of tragedy of the loss. This will help put things in perspective.

The meaning of a score of one should be some small thing, such as a stubbed toe. The meaning of a score of one hundred would be something tragic such as nuclear war or the death of a loved one. The meaning of the score of fifty is somewhere in between a stubbed toe and nuclear war. In all three of these scores, the meaning should be up to you. You may feel a stubbed toe is more like a twenty and going to your in-laws for a weekend is one hundred. My examples are only to give you a sense of the extremes.

Once you define the scale, plot where your loss falls. Does it feel like it's a sixty? Or does it feel like a twenty? If we are honest, most losses and underperformances we experience do not constitute tragedy like a nuclear war. So, by putting your loss on such a scale, you can quickly move past any level one or level two thoughts you might have about your loss.

Once you can cope with the loss, you will be ready to move to the next stage: finding the gift.

STEP 2: Find the gift (the servant). The second step is to ask yourself what gift will come from the loss or under performance. This probably seems the last question you will want to entertain after a loss. How you can win and beat your opponent are usually the questions you ask the most. However, to put yourself in a strong position to win again, you do need to get your mindset up to a high level again. Finding the gift from the loss is a part of that process.

For spiritual people, this is a time to pray and reflect. You might need to journal a little bit. Try free-zone journaling or writing, or just talking aloud. You may need the help of a coach to help you probe and find the gift.

After some reflection, you may find the gift. For instance, maybe there's a weakness in your game that needs improvement. By working on that part of your game, you can elevate your skills and be in a strong position to win the next time around. Whatever the gift might be, what is important is to experience gratitude for the gift and embrace it genuinely.

STEP 3: Find the opportunity (the opportunist). The third and final step is to identify the learning from the loss. Ask yourself, "What can I learn from this experience? What else might this experience be presenting to me?"

For many athletes, this is often what you do with your coaches after you regroup from a loss. What is important in this step, however, is to approach learning from a genuine place of curiosity and non-judgment. A level three (rationalizer), mindset can often mask itself by trying to cope with the loss under the guise of learning. That is why completing steps one and two can be so important for getting into this mindset: they clear the judgment you may be placing on the experience.

Often, the opportunity comes right off of step two and perfects it: you may realize you have a hole in your game that needs to be patched up and now the opportunity is to develop that skill and patch up the hole. Once you have identified the learning opportunity, you will likely experience some excitement and/or peace about the experience. This is a sign you are viewing the loss from an opportunist mindset.

Once you've found the learning element, immediately work with your coach to embed the learning into your muscle memory so your skill and technique can immediately improve for the next game. By doing this on a regular basis, you will drastically improve your skills and your overall enjoyment of your sport.

As you work with this three-stage process, you can gradually alter and condense the practice into a quick trigger that allows you to immediately transform any loss into a powerful performance-improvement tool. Over time, you will see losses phase you less and less and your skill grow to such high levels that you put yourself in fewer positions to lose.

Key Points

- Losing can be a powerful detractor from getting in the zone and can affect future performances.
- The first step to handing a loss is to cope with it by putting it into the bigger picture. Plotting the loss on a scale of one to one hundred to see whether it's truly a tragedy or not will help you determine how you choose to let this affect you.
- The second step to handling a loss is to find the gift in the situation.
- The third step to dealing with a loss is to find the learning from the situation and grow from it.

chapter

7

Zone Inhibitor: Injury

"Our greatest weakness lies in giving up.
The most certain way to succeed is always to try just one more time."
THOMAS EDISON

NOTHING IS DREADED MORE by athletes than becoming injured during the season, whether this happens during preparation training or during the competition season. Missing competitions and sitting on the sidelines is the last experience any athlete is looking to have in their season. Beyond the physical impact of injury, your mindset can suffer. You can feel like you've lost your edge and doubt, fear, and worry can creep in.

From a mindset perspective, you will likely experience one of three (if not all) mindsets during injury.

The first is the victim mindset. In this mindset, you feel like the injury happened to you and you have no power over the situation. You are at the mercy of the injury until it gets better. Being in this mindset is the lowest level of energy and engagement you can have within your life and sport. However, it can also be the most difficult to detect, and you may never want to admit you are experiencing it. Nonetheless, symptoms of this mindset include dragging your feet, feeling heavy, replaying the event over and over in your mind, and feeling bad that you are missing time away from your team.

The second is the aggressor mindset. At this level, you may be feeling angry at yourself, someone else, and the situation of being injured. Detecting this mindset is much easier than the victim mindset. However, it still is a catabolic-energy-based mindset and will keep you from your highest potential in the long run. It also releases stress hormones such as cortisol in your body, which can delay the healing process.

The third is the rationalizer mindset. At this level, you will have moved beyond the victim and aggressor mindsets and will focus on coping with the circumstances. The coping process involves looking at the situation from the standpoint of doing the best you can, finding something positive to focus on, and forgiving yourself and others. It is a major step in the process of facing injury. However, you won't want to remain here too long if you are to heal quickly and get back into the game.

So, you might ask, what can I do to improve the situation?

Getting the Mindset Back

STEP 1: Acceptance. Acceptance may be a difficult process for you because accepting something like injury can seem like weakness. Nonetheless, finding a way to accept the situation will lessen the catabolic energy that is associated with the victim and aggressor mindsets (if you are experiencing these mindsets). To do this, write a definition of acceptance around the injury and repeat it. You might write something like this:

I choose to accept that I am, for the moment, physically injured and unable to train and compete the way I would like. However, I know this isn't the worst thing in the world or the end of my career. I let go of any fear, worry, doubt, anger, or victim feelings. I choose to experience peace in this situation because I know everything works to make me a better athlete.

By defining your version of acceptance of the situation and practicing it, you will give yourself power over the situation and put yourself in the driver's seat again. You will create a 'space' between the stimulus and response, which will allow you to return to the eye of the hurricane.

STEP 2: Find the gift and serve (servant mindset—level four). This is a mirror to step two in the earlier chapter on loss. Ask yourself, "What might the gift be here?" You may need to take a few reflection sessions or discuss this with your coach, teammate, friend, or partner. Eventually, the answer will present itself to you.

Further, if you are in a team sport, you can boost your mindset by showing up to serve your team during their practices. This may take the form of encouraging them, spotting them during strength and conditioning workouts, or any other forms of support you can provide for them. If you are not in a team sport, find a way to support a friend, family member, or partner in some way. By serving someone, you will move outside yourself and forget about your injury for a while.

STEP 3: Focus on the learning and fun (opportunist mindset – level five). What might you have learned from this situation? Take time to actively think about it. Your lessons may be something directly related to the game or more about life itself. Some athletes find that injuries are critical times where they can reinvent their game and add to their toolkit. In any case, finding lessons that you can feel peace and excitement about are important for keeping your mindset at a higher level during injury.

Find ways to have fun. I don't mean reckless partying; I mean find some way to keep your spirits high and your mindset off the injury. You might want to combine the servant mindset and opportunist mindsets by organizing a team party or team event that everyone can enjoy. You may want to combine your lessons with some fun. For instance, if you learned that your shooting technique puts too much stress on your knees, you might decide to have a fun practice. Whatever you choose to do, don't forget to have some fun along the way.

In short, the overall strategy for dealing with injuries from a mental perspective is to take the power back. To get out of a victim, aggressor, or rationalizer mindset and put yourself back in a state of learning.

To further the process of taking your power back, there is an additional mindset strategy you can follow.

Keeping Skills Sharp, Even While Being Injured

Visualization is a powerful tool for continuing to take back your power. Even though you may not be able to train at your previous levels, you can keep your skills sharp through visualization.

There is a famous study of basketball players that tested the effect of visualization on their free-throw accuracy. In this study, conducted by Dr. Biasiotto at the University of Chicago, three groups of players were tested on the impacts of different training methods on free-throw accuracy. Group A shot free throws for one hour each day; Group B just visualized themselves shooting free throws (and making each one every time); Group C did nothing. After thirty days, Dr. Biasiotto tested each group. The results are telling:[43]

- Group A: 24% improvement in making free throws.
- Group B: 23% improvement in making free throws.
- Group C: No improvement.

The results of this study strongly suggest that visualization, when done correctly, can improve your motor skills almost as well as actual practice.

Of course, the results do not suggest you should just visualize and not practice if you are healthy. However, the results do offer a lot of consolation for the injured athlete looking to keep their skills and mindset sharp while injured.

To put visualization to practice for yourself while injured, follow these steps below.

STEP 1: Identify the movements. Work with your coach to identify the key movements, skills, and game plans you need to keep fresh and sharp. It may be free-throw shots for a basketball player, tackles for a football player, striking for a combat athlete, or swings for a golfer.

STEP 2: For each movement and game plan, visualize yourself executing it for five minutes or more (timing for each will depend on how many you have to perform). Use vivid imagery that engages all of your senses (smell, taste, feel, sight, and hearing). The more you engage your senses, the more the imagery is engrained in your neural networks.

STEP 3: Visualize with certainty. In addition to engaging all your senses, be sure to see the execution of each movement or game plan with certainty. If you are practicing free throws, see the shots sink each time. If you are practicing striking, see each strike land with maximum effect on your opponent. Spend at least one hour a day in visualization. It will keep your neural networks as fresh as possible and help you keep your sense of power over your situation stronger.

VISUALIZATION TIP ONE: practice in a quiet place where you won't be distracted. It is important to allow yourself the chance to enter into the visualization without distraction.

VISUALIZATION TIP TWO: you can enhance your experience by listening to binaural beat music. Binaural beat music entrains your brain into a targeted brainwave (see chapter two) by playing different frequencies into each ear, the difference of which equals the target brain frequency (e.g., 480 hz in left ear and 468 hz in the right ear; the difference being 12 hz, the alpha brain-wave frequency). Targeting a theta (3 – 8 hz) or alpha

(8 – 14 hz) brain-wave state for visualization will help ensure your brain absorbs the impact of the training to maximum effect. Alpha and theta binaural beat music can be found on the Internet for free.

VISUALIZATION TIP THREE: sensory deprivation tanks can provide a powerful benefit for visualization by combining tips one and two. In a sensory deprivation tank, you float in a quiet tank of water (water is denser due to Epsom salt mixture that ensures you float), which provides a quiet place free of distractions and will allow your mind to enter into a theta brain state. Additional benefits include relaxation and faster recovery (even from your injury).

Starting to Train After Injury

Even if you have been cleared to return to training and competition by a doctor, you may still experience mindset challenges. While most trainers, doctors, and coaches will have you ease back into training (as you should), your mindset can sometimes hold you back even though you are ready to be 100%. Often you can experience doubts such as "What if I re-injure myself?" These doubts lead to playing cautiously and lower your performance.

One strategy you can use to quell some of these doubts is to give yourself pleasure-based rewards for completing training activities in the area of the injury. For instance, as a basketball player, if you sprained your ankle while performing a jump shot, you may want to start practicing jump shots at twenty percent of your average intensity. For each you perform, you might give yourself your favorite candy or get a kiss from your partner (reward). As you gain comfort at twenty-percent intensity, you can increase to fifty percent, eighty percent, and then to 100% following the same reward system.

By gradually increasing the intensity and providing yourself with a pleasurable reward after successful completion at each intensity level, you will establish a positive neural connection with the activity that was previously associated with the injury. As a result, you can break the fear and worry that might have been related to using the part of your body that was injured. (See the chapter on fear and worry for guidance in handling these emotions).

Key Points

- Injury can dramatically affect your mindset by putting you into a victim, aggressor, or rationalizer mindset.
- You can take your power back, even during an injury, by taking control of your mindset.
- Practicing gratitude and focusing on learning and fun can help keep your mindset in a high state.
- Practicing visualization can keep your skills sharp while you are injured. Visualize your key movements with certainty and using all your senses.
- To move past any potential worry of re-injuring yourself when you come back (once you are medically cleared), gradually increase the intensity of usage and provide yourself a reward each time you perform the movement.

chapter

8

Zone Inhibitor: Losing Motivation

"Optimism is the faith that leads to achievement. Nothing can be done without hope and confidence."
HELEN KELLER

MOTIVATION IS ONE OF THE KEYS to peak performance. You know all too well what happens when you lose motivation. Your interest goes down. Your performance goes down. You stop enjoying your sport as much. For a professional athlete (and those aspiring to be so), these consequences can have serious effects on your career. For non-professionals, these consequences are the last experience you want to have, given the free time you are giving up for your sport.

Basketball, hockey and baseball players have long seasons. Baseball players play over one hundred and sixty games. Basketball and hockey players over eighty games. Football players have sixteen intense games (counting all the hits taken). Soccer players have over thirty games (considering all of the stamina required for their games). Endurance athletes have rigorous training, taking place over six months leading up to the main event. Combat sports athletes train two to three times a day at high intensity in preparation for their fights. It can get repetitious and tiring. In addition, if you aren't seeing the desired results, it is easy to lose motivation.

So, it makes sense you would ask: how do you keep your motivation high, especially during long seasons, hard training, and discouraging results?

Types of Motivation

The first phase to keeping your motivation high is understanding the types of motivation available to you. There are two types of motivation: intrinsic motivation and extrinsic motivation.

Intrinsic motivation is doing something for the fun of it, for the enjoyment of it, for its own sake with little thought as to what you get from the experience. Examples of intrinsic motivation are playing baseball for the love of the game, fighting for the love of fighting, playing basketball for the love of basketball, and competing for the enjoyment of it. It's simply the satisfaction derived from just doing the activity itself.

Extrinsic motivation is doing an activity for the external reward it will produce. For instance, becoming an endurance athlete so you can have a fit body; doing conditioning work so you can have a beach body; becoming a professional basketball player to make lots of money or obtain celebrity status; or wanting to win the championship so you can have bragging rights. These are extrinsic motivators.

Both will produce motivation and are neither good nor bad. They just *are*. However, what you will notice with extrinsic motivation is that if you don't get the results you desire, your levels of motivation can wane.

Intrinsic motivation, on the other hand, can keep you going. It's a powerful fuel. You can renew it all the time. You can *always* have fun. You can *always* do something for the enjoyment of the activity itself. The real strategy around motivation is to tap into intrinsic motivation on a consistent basis.

Boosting Motivation

Boosting motivation does not necessarily following a step-by-step process. Instead, I've identified several considerations for you to review. As you review each, see which considerations may be applicable for you in your situation right now. You can incorporate one or all of these considerations. Each will help your motivation levels.

CONSIDERATION 1: Focus on intrinsic goals. Now that you see the two types of motivation available to you, it is important to have at least one goal that is oriented to intrinsic motivation. This means looking to be involved for reasons connected to the love of the sport and game. This might involve how you feel after your workout, the enjoyment of your teammates company, and how great it feels to flawlessly execute a move (or master a new one).

To set goals based on intrinsic motivation, consider the parts of the game you initially fell in love with. Once you have identified these elements, create at least one goal for yourself based on these elements. Your goal may be simply to have fun each day of practice and competitions. On the other hand, you may want to focus on experiencing the elements of the sport you initially fell in love with.

CONSIDERATION 2: Develop a morning power ritual. A ritual is a regular practice to achieve a specific purpose; in this case, giving yourself motivation every morning (it may or may not involve religion, depending on your beliefs). A morning power ritual is one of the first priorities you should set for yourself every morning to ensure you keep your motivation levels high.

Tony Robbins, a world-renowned life and business strategist, recommends a session lasting between fifteen minutes to one hour, calling them 'fifteen minutes to fulfillment,' 'thirty minutes to thrive,' or an 'an hour of power.' A key component of his morning rituals involves a threefold approach: energize your emotions, focus, and language patterns (common questions and phrases you use) by following a routine of breathing exercises, practicing gratitude, visualization, and incantations while you are walking.[44]

To develop your morning power ritual, consider following this sample structure. Each of these items will energize your emotions, set your focus on the right step, and help you develop powerful language patterns.

> **Gratitude:** Identify three (or more) things you are grateful for in your life each morning. Take five minutes or more to bring each item to your mind and heart. Be sure to see, feel, and hear each item and the gratitude you have for each item.
>
> **Visualization:** Visualize the accomplishment of your season goals (and life goals if you'd like). Take five minutes or more to see, feel, and hear the achievement of each goal. Be sure to bring to mind the emotions you identified in step one.
>
> **Incantations/Affirmations:** Incantations/affirmations are brief phrases you repeat aloud that engrain a specific belief into your subconscious mind. For instance, "I am unstoppable" or "I can do all things I put my mind to." Develop one short phrase that strikes you as powerful. Then repeat it aloud for five minutes or more. The more emotion you put into it, the better.
>
> **Walking/running/other physical activity:** You might want to go for a walk or run in the morning. Alternatively, you can do sit-ups and pushups or some other moderate activity. This gets your blood flowing and boosts your metabolism. Depending on your workout, this may fit into your schedule.
>
> **Journaling:** You may find journaling briefly in the morning to

be a helpful activity. You might journal about what you are grateful for and write down some of your visualizations. You also might want to write down your incantations. Or you may choose to write down what you want to accomplish for the day.

TIP #1
You can combine the HeartMath breathing technique (see chapter five) with gratitude and visualization.

TIP #2
You can practice incantations/affirmations in front of the mirror. The mirror technique is a powerful way to engrain the specific belief into your subconscious mind.[45]

CONSIDERATION 3: "Identify motivation blocks. Take some time to reflect on your internal sources. These sources of that drain motivation come from within:"[46]

Bodily – Are you tired from lots of training, competing, and travel? Lack of sleep? Lack of adequate nutrition and hydration?

Emotional – Are you feeling catabolic emotions such as anger, frustration, annoyance, lethargy, or others like these?

Mental – Are you feeling overwhelmed by so many distractions and too many things on your to-do list?

Purpose – Are you living according to your sense of purpose?

External sources. These sources of that drain motivation come from around you:

People – Are people around you draining you? Do you have the right ratio of time alone vs. time with people?

Environment – Is the weather de-motivating you? Is the equipment you are using for your sport optimal for you? Is your routine confining you?

Once you have identified the blocks at work, you can devise ways to boost your motivation. For instance, if your body is tired, get the rest and nutrition you need. If you are emotionally tired, then practice anabolic emotions (levels four – seven). If you are drained by the people around you, then spend more time alone or get around people who motivate you.

Key Points

- Motivation is key to getting in and staying in the zone. However, your training and competing schedule can often get in the way of your motivation levels.

- There are two types of motivation: intrinsic and extrinsic motivation. Intrinsic motivation is the enjoyment of the sport in of itself; extrinsic motivation is enjoyment of the victories, awards, publicity, etc. from your sport.

- You can rely and increase on intrinsic motivation because it is always within your power; extrinsic motivation depends on things not directly within your power (e.g. winning).

- You can sustain intrinsic motivation by setting and focusing goals that are within your control and are enjoyable (e.g. learning, having fun).

- You can boost daily motivation by developing a morning power ritual that involves any combination of practicing gratitude, visualization, physical activity, and journaling.

- You can also raise motivation by identifying the source of its drainage—bodily, emotional, mental, purpose, social, and environmental sources.

chapter

9

The Seven Levels of Performance Process

MY DESIRE FOR YOU IS that this book has provided you with some practical tips you can immediately implement into your sport that will translate into immediate results. Getting into the zone can seem like such an elusive process, and not having the right resources for understanding how to make this happen can be a real block. I know when I was competing, I wish I'd had a guidebook like this one to help me along the way.

Not getting into the zone on a consistent basis can hold you back. This can mean the difference between winning and losing, having your best financial payouts or not, winning the championship or not, being sponsored or not, making the team or not, being drafted or not, and enjoying your sport or not.

Whether you are a professional, aspiring professional, or hobbyist athlete, getting into the zone gives you the edge. The seven levels of performance provide the understanding of mindset so you can shift your mindset into higher levels, which means getting into the zone.

If you are enjoying The Seven Levels of Performance and finding yourself wondering which levels you tend to frequent in your sport and life, there is a way to find out. The Seven Levels of Performance process includes a power assessment for identifying these levels. This assessment from iPEC, called Energy Leadership Assessment (ELI)™, will show you a few key aspects of your mindset:

- Mindset under normal conditions: your primary, secondary, and tertiary mindsets you have in life and your sport when things are going well for you. This will allow you to see where you can still shift your mindset in order to experience the zone.

- Mindset under stress: your primary, secondary, and tertiary mindsets you have in life and your sport when you experience a stress reaction (anything that triggers you like fatigue, a referee call you disagree with, etc.). This will show you the greatest opportunity for improvement in your mindset because these stress reactions will prevent you from being in the zone and/or taking you out of the zone.

- Key beliefs that may be holding you back from experiencing the zone on a more consistent basis.

I have yet to see another assessment which covers the scope of mindset like this. Most people who take it find it to be accurate and insightful.

If you would like to learn more about this assessment and how you can take it, visit my website at www.chrismorganlive.com/services/assessment-process.

When deciding whether to take the assessment or not, the critical factor is realizing what option you are aligned with. What is your clear "yes" and what is your clear "no."

If you find yourself enjoying this material and think it can help your athletic career, this may indicate a *yes*. However, if you feel this is not the support you need at this time, this may indicate a *no*.

In either event, my hope is that you find what works for you in getting you into the zone on a more consistent basis so you can have your best performances and enjoy your sport the most.

To that hope, I repeat the opening quote of the book: "Good, better and best. Never rest, 'til your good is better, and your better is best."

—Chris Morgan

Bonus:
Six Principles of the Zone

Getting in the zone consistently gives you the edge. It involves mental toughness but ends up going well beyond it because it makes performance seem effortless, timeless, creative, and awesome. So that means having your best and most enjoyable performances. And that can define your legacy.

In my work helping teams and individuals experience peak performance more consistently, I've found a collection of about six principles that characterize the way athletes and other peak performers get into the zone on a consistent basis. I've studied loads of peak performance systems and these principles can be found in these systems as well. These six principles, when practiced regularly, can help you get in, and stay in, the zone more consistently.

You can get this one-sheet reminder as my gift to you. Post where it will help nudge your thinking and encourage you to make every performance solid. Go here to get your free tip sheet: ChrisMorganLive.com

Will You Please Leave A Review?

I'D BE GRATEFUL IF you'd leave a review on Amazon. People benefit from your input and make decisions based on what people like you have to say. When they purchase, of course I benefit a bit from the income on books, but what I cherish the most is having the book make a difference in people's lives. Your review might be the one that makes that happen. Thanks in advance for doing so.

References

1. Herculano-Houzel, Suzanne. *"The Human Brain in Numbers: A Linearly Scaled-up Primate Brain"*. https://www.ncbi.nlm.nih.gov/pmc/articles/PMC2776484/

2. Schneider, Bruce D. *"Energy Leadership."* Pg. 12

3. Based on iPEC Coach Training

4. Schneider, Bruce D. *"Energy Leadership."* Pg. 16

5. Ibid., Pg. 13

6. Kotler, Steven. *"The Rise of Superman."* Pgs. 68 - 69

7. Ibid., Pgs. 49 - 51

8. Ibid., Pg. 51

9. HeartMath, *"HeartMath Brain Fitness Program"*. Pg. 14 - 16

10. Oxford Reference, *"Inverted U Hypothesis"*. http://www.oxfordreference.com/view/10.1093/oi/authority.20110803100009722

11. Csikszentmihalyi, Mihaly. *"Flow."* Pgs. 49 - 67

12. Robbins, Tony. Online source.

13. Mumford, George. *"The Mindful Athlete."* Pg., 71

14. Gracie, Rickson. Online social media source

15. Waitzkin, Josh. *"The Art of Learning"*. Pg. 190

16. Ibid., pgs. 188 - 190

17. Ibid., pg. 194

18. Ibid., pg 194

19. Rock, David. *"Your Brain at Work"*. Pg. 151

20. Ibid., Pg. 151

21. Based on the MeartMath breathing technique, *"HeartMath Brain Fitness Program"* Pg. 78 (e-book version)

22 Ibid., Pg. 137

23 Ibid., Pg. 138

24 Ibid., Pg. 143

25 Ibid., Pg. 145

26 *Star Wars: Episode VI*

27 Gracie, Rener and Ririon. Online social media video

28 Coyle, Daniel. *"The Talent Code."* Pg. 32.

29 Ibid., Pg. 33

30 Ibid., Pg. 18

31 Ibid., Pgs. 79 – 94

32 Ibid., Pg. 88

33 Ibid., Pg. 92

34 Ibid., Pg. 53

35 Mumford, George. *"The Mindful Athlete."* Pg., 96

36 Ibid., Pg.107

37 Devine, Mark. *"The Way of the Seal."* Pgs. 100 – 102

38 Ibid., Pg. 100

39 Ibid., Pg. 100

40 HearthMath Brain Fitness Program. Pg., 78 (e-book version)

41 Devine, Mark. *"The Way of the Seal."* Pg. 101

42 Robbins, Tony. Online source.

43 Haefner, Joe. Mental Rehearsal and Visualization. https://www.breakthroughbasketball.com/mental/visualization.html

44 Robbins, Tony. *"The Edge."* (audio book)

45 Bristol, Clause, M. *"The Magic Of Believing"*

46 Concepts derived from iPEC COR.E Dynamics Program, *"The Six Energy Influencers"*

If you'd like to order
bulk copies (25 or more)
for gifts and/or for a team,
please contact
admin@ThePublishingCircle.com
for special pricing.

www.ChrisMorganLive.com

www.ingramcontent.com/pod-product-compliance
Lightning Source LLC
Chambersburg PA
CBHW060032040426
42333CB00042B/2405